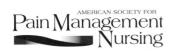 AMERICAN SOCIETY FOR
Pain Management
Nursing

D0947385

 IA
NURSES
ATION

Pain Management Nursing:

Scope and Standards
of Practice

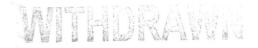

nurses
books
.org
The Publishing Program of ANA

American Nurses Association
Silver Spring, MD
2005

Library of Congress Cataloging-in-Publication data

American Society for Pain Management Nursing.
  Pain management nursing : scope and standards of practice / American Society for Pain Management Nursing [and] American Nurses Association.
      p. ; cm.
  Includes bibliographical references and index.
  ISBN-13: 978-1-55810-226-2
  ISBN-10: 1-55810-226-4
  1. Pain—Nursing. 2. Pain—Nursing—Standards.
  [DNLM: 1. Pain—nursing. 2. Nursing Assessment—standards. 3. Nursing Care—standards. WY 160.5 A5126 2005] I. American Nurses Association. II. Title.

  RT87.P35.A447 2005
  616.07'5—dc22   2005005495

The American Nurses Association (ANA) is a national professional association. This ANA publication—*Pain Management Nursing: Scope and Standards of Practice*—reflects the thinking of the nursing profession on various issues and should be reviewed in conjunction with state board of nursing policies and practices. State law, rules, and regulations govern the practice of nursing, while *Pain Management Nursing: Scope and Standards of Practice* guides nurses in the application of their professional skills and responsibilities.

The American Society for Pain Management Nursing is an organization of professional nurses. The Society's mission is to advance and promote optimal nursing care for people affected by pain.

Published by nursesbooks.org
The Publishing Program of ANA

American Nurses Association
8515 Georgia Avenue, Suite 400
Silver Spring, MD 20910-3492
1-800-274-4ANA
http://www.nursesbooks.org/

ANA is the only full-service professional organization representing the nation's 2.7 million Registered Nurses through its 54 constituent member associations. ANA advances the nursing profession by fostering high standards of nursing practice, promoting the economic and general welfare of nurses in the workplace, projecting a positive and realistic view of nursing, and lobbying the Congress and regulatory agencies on healthcare issues affecting nurses and the public.

ISBN 978-1-55810-226-2   05SSPM   2M   12/06R

First printing April 2005. Second printing December 2006.

CONTENTS

ACKNOWLEDGMENTS

The Standards of Clinical Nursing Practice for Pain Management have undergone several revisions over the years, culminating in *Pain Management Nursing: Scope and Standards of Practice*. The efforts of many members of the American Society for Pain Management Nursing are reflected in this work.

Scope and Standards Task Force
Georgette Love, MSN, APRN, *Chair*
Catherine Beattie, MS, RN, CNA
Micke Brown, BSN, RN,C
Theresa A. Grimes, MN, RN, FNP-C, CCRN
Mary Heye, PhD, RN, CS
Michael Ann Pandolph, MS, RN, ANP, OCN
Joan D. Wentz, MSN, RN, CS, ANP

Scope and Standards Revision Task Force
Theresa A. Grimes, MN, RN, FNP-C, CCRN
Joan D. Wentz, MSN, RN, CS, ANP
Barbara St. Marie, MA, RN, CS, ANP, GNP

Expert Reviewers
Christine Miaskowski, PhD, RN, FAAN
Barbara Reed, MN, RN, CGNP
Susan Pendergrass, MSN, MEd, RN, CS, FNP
Barbara Urbanski, MS, RN

Staff
Belinda E. Puetz, PhD, RN
Patricia M. Barlow

ANA Staff
Carol Bickford, PhD, RN,BC – *Content Editor*
Yvonne Humes, MSA
Winifred Carson, JD

INTRODUCTION

Pain is the most common nursing diagnosis in all delivery-of-care models; therefore, the assessment and management of pain is within the purview of every professional registered nurse (RN). In a U.S. survey in July 2003, 57% of respondents had experienced chronic persistent pain over the previous year (Researchamerica.org 2003). As pervasive as these statistics are, many people, including residents in healthcare facilities, minority groups, and patients across the life span, continue to be undertreated for painful procedures and conditions. The undertreatment of pain drove research that led the International Association for the Study of Pain (IASP) to define pain as "an unpleasant sensory and emotional experience associated with actual or potential tissue damage, or described in terms of such damage" (Merskey 1979).

The incidence of pain, regardless of healthcare environment or age group, prompted a group of nurses to discuss their unique role in improving these statistics. In 1990 they dedicated themselves to developing pain management nursing based on scientific evidence, a theoretical framework, and core practices consistent with the American Nurses Association (ANA) *Scope of Nursing Practice* (1987). This groundwork focused on comprehensive pain management to foster optimal physical function and quality of life for all patients with pain.

Theoretic constructs have provided the framework on which pain management nursing is built today. René Descartes first described pain anatomically in 1644. His simplistic model described a one-way afferent pathway of transmission "like pulling of a thread" from a foot embedded in fire to the awareness of pain occurring in the brain. In 1896 this theory was further expanded by Max von Frey, who identified specific receptors throughout the body that were sensitive to pain, temperature, and touch. Von Frey's specificity theory described receptors that responded to specific stimuli and transmitted a specific signal along a specific nerve to a specific part of the brain (Rey 1993). Other theories followed, such as the Gate Control Theory and the Pattern Theory, developed by Melzack and Wall (1965, 1983). These theories were the first to consider the psychological and emotional aspects of pain, and are used in modern pain management practices.

Recent strides in pain research have detailed multifaceted interactions of transduction, transmission, perception, and modulation of acute, chronic (persistent), and neuropathic pain that are beyond the scope of this document. The reader is referred to the American Society of Pain Management

Nurses (ASPMN) *Core Curriculum for Pain Management Nursing* (St. Marie 2002) which synthesizes several scientific works into a theoretical framework.

"A knowledge base has developed that includes the physical, social, cultural, psychological, and spiritual dimensions of the pain experience" (ASPMN 1997). As a result of this knowledge base and current pain research, a unique set of terms has emerged to describe the experience of pain. Terms such as somatosensory, visceral, and neuropathic describe the origin of pain; allodynia and hyperalgesia describe the perception of pain; and pain and suffering are distinguished and treated as specific entities and not simply symptoms. Medication management for pain syndromes has led to new definitions of tolerance, dependence, addiction, and pseudoaddiction. Furthermore, guidelines and standards for pain management have been developed by organizations such as the Agency for Healthcare Research and Quality (AHRQ) (Carr et al. 1992; Jacox et al. 1994; Welsh et al. 2000), the American Pain Society (APS) (Ashburn et al. 2003; Benjamin et al. 1999; Max et al. 1998; Payne et al. 1997; Simon et al. 1999, 2002), the Joint Commission on Accreditation of Healthcare Organizations (JCAHO), the Federation of State Boards of Medicine, and the American Society of Pain Management Nurses (ASPMN) (1996, 1997, 1998).

Some key elements of *Pain Management Nursing: Scope and Standards of Practice* incorporate interdisciplinary approaches to pain management offered in a variety of healthcare settings. Other elements include understanding pathophysiology of pain, and techniques for improving pain relief, optimizing function, and maintaining quality of life.

The role of the nurse generalist and the nurse specialist is supported through these Standards of Practice, adapted from the foundational American Nurses Association publication, *Nursing: Scope and Standards of Practice* (2004). The nurse generalist is provided with standards of practice designed to provide comprehensive pain management knowledge and skills throughout the nursing process, supported by evidence-based practice as found in the *Core Curriculum for Pain Management Nursing* (St. Marie 2002). The nurse specialist in pain management has mastered a body of knowledge in pain management, incorporates this body of knowledge into clinical practice regardless of setting, and synthesizes the multidimensional aspects of pain and the varied individual responses to pain influenced by age, gender, culture, or socioeconomic status. Pain management nurse specialists advocate resolving ethical issues of patients, colleagues, or systems involving pain management as defined by *Code of Ethics for Nurses with Interpretive Statements* (ANA 2001) and Greipp's Model for Ethical Decision Making (Greipp 1992).

To further safeguard individuals and ensure professional accountability for pain management, ASPMN has released several position statements addressing such things as the use of placebos, pain management in patients with addictive disease, neonatal circumcision pain relief, assisted suicide, and end-of-life care. In addition, ASPMN has published clinical practice guidelines on geriatric pain assessment, patient-controlled analgesia, and epidural analgesia to assist the nurse generalist and pain management nurse specialist in their practices.

As scientific theories in pain management nursing continue to evolve, further issues of formalizing educational endeavors need to be addressed, such as credentialing nurses in pain management practice. Presently, formal education in pain management at the advanced practice level is incorporated into Master's Education in Palliative Care programs and in efforts of the End-of-Life Nurse Educators Consortium (ELNEC). Universal incorporation of pain management across a basic nursing curriculum is in the future.

Cancer pain initiatives and state pain initiatives have evolved into advocacy for all patients in pain. These efforts will help drive practice and foster developments in pain management. Furthermore, the National Institutes of Health has established a National Center for Pain and Palliative Care Research to promote optimal pain management based on nursing and medical research.

Pain management nursing is an ongoing, dynamic process. Nurses have incorporated pain management into myriad roles, including but not limited to caregiver, patient advocate, educator, change agent, manager, clinical nurse specialist, nurse practitioner, and researcher. In 2003, the American Nurses Credentialing Center (ANCC) approved the certification process for pain management nursing based on the *Core Curriculum for Pain Management Nursing* (St. Marie 2002) and clinical performance. The following pages are a basis for operationalizing the Core's theoretical framework into practice and establishing a minimum standard of pain management nursing practice.

Standards of Pain Management Nursing: Standards of Practice

Standard 1. Assessment

The registered nurse collects comprehensive data pertinent to the pain problem.

Standard 2. Diagnosis

The registered nurse analyzes the assessment data to determine pain diagnoses or problems.

Standard 3. Outcomes Identification

The registered nurse identifies expected pain management outcomes for a plan individualized to the patient with pain.

Standard 4. Planning

The registered nurse develops a pain management plan that prescribes strategies and alternatives to attain expected outcomes.

Standard 5. Implementation

The registered nurse implements the identified pain management plan.

Standard 5a: Coordination of Care

The registered nurse coordinates the pain management plan.

Standard 5b: Health Teaching and Health Promotion

The registered nurse employs strategies to promote, maintain, and restore pain-relieving behaviors.

Standard 5c: Consultation

The advanced practice registered nurse provides consultation to influence the identified pain management plan, enhance the abilities of others, and effect change.

Standard 5d: Prescriptive Authority and Treatment

The advanced practice registered nurse uses prescriptive authority, procedures, referrals, treatments, and therapies in accordance with state and federal laws and regulations.

Standard 6. Evaluation

The registered nurse evaluates progress towards attainment of acceptable pain management outcomes.

Standards of Pain Management Nursing: Standards of Professional Performance

Standard 7. Quality of Practice
The registered nurse systematically evaluates the quality and effectiveness of pain management practice.

Standard 8. Education
The registered nurse attains knowledge and competency that reflects current pain management nursing practice.

Standard 9. Professional Practice Evaluation
The registered nurse evaluates their own nursing practice in relation to professional pain practice standards and guidelines, relevant statutes, rules, and regulations.

Standard 10. Collegiality
The registered nurse interacts with, and contributes to the professional development of, peers and colleagues.

Standard 11. Collaboration
The registered nurse collaborates with patient, family, and others in the conduct of pain management nursing practice.

Standard 12. Ethics
The registered nurse integrates ethical provisions to guide pain management practices.

Standard 13. Research
The registered nurse integrates pain research findings into clinical practice.

Standard 14. Resource Utilization
The registered nurse considers factors related to safety, effectiveness, cost, and impact on practice in the planning and delivery of pain management.

Standard 15. Leadership
The registered nurse provides leadership in professional pain management.

SCOPE OF PRACTICE OF PAIN MANAGEMENT NURSING

Pain management nursing is the application of nursing practice based on scientific principles aimed at alleviating pain and suffering in patients in a variety of healthcare settings. Pharmacological and non-pharmacological nursing interventions eliminate or reduce the pain that results in diminished quality of life. The science of pain, and pain itself, are dynamic and constantly changing. Thus, pain management nursing must accommodate these changes. In response to the growing need for nurses with scientific knowledge and demonstrated clinical expertise related to pain management, the American Society for Pain Management Nursing (ASPMN) has sought formal recognition as a nursing specialty from the American Nurses Association and has established a specialty certification examination to be first offered in October 2005.

History

Evidence-based theory and practice for nurses influencing the management of patients' pain began in 1960 at the University of Washington in Seattle, and at the City of Hope in Duarte, California, where nurses were employed in pain clinics. In 1962 the National League for Nursing funded a project at the University of California at Los Angeles that resulted in the first book and an accompanying film, both titled *Pain and Its Alleviation,* written and produced by a nurse, Dorothy M. Crowley. This was followed in 1967 by a classic article written by Ada Rogers that identified the basic information nurses need to successfully titrate analgesics for cancer pain management. Margo McCaffery published a clinical definition of pain, which is the cornerstone of pain assessment today: "Pain is whatever the experiencing person says it is, existing whenever he says it does" (1968, 195).

In the 1970s, the nursing profession responded to these pain nurse pioneers by including separate chapters in nursing textbooks that focused on pain management. McCaffery continued to champion nursing pain management with the publication of *Nursing Management of the Patient with Pain* (1972, 1979). *Pain: A Source Book for Nurses and Other Health Professionals*, edited by Ada Jacox, was published in 1977. Jacox and Mary Steward also published a monograph of their research on the patient's total pain experience in 1978.

The International Association for the Study of Pain (IASP) was founded with the help of nurses in 1974. In 1977 IASP approved chapter status for the

American Pain Society (APS) with several nurses as founding members. The first edition of the APS *Principles of Analgesic Use* (Payne et al. 1987) was published with the assistance of nurses who served as committee members and reviewers.

The Nursing Pain Association became the first pain specialty nursing organization in 1987. Composed of nurse clinicians and researchers, this association made its primary goal to link research in pain to clinical practice (Pasero 2003). The first extensive, research-based textbook for the nursing care of patients with pain was published by two nurses (McCaffery and Beebe 1989; McCaffery and Pasero 1999). Nurses also helped the World Health Organization revise its publication *Cancer Pain Relief and Palliative Care* in 1990.

The American Society of Pain Management Nurses, now the American Society for Pain Management Nursing (ASPMN), was founded in 1990 by a small group of nurses interested in providing better pain management to patients. Since then ASPMN has grown into a large organization of committed nurses with the same goal as the charter membership. ASPMN supports nurses who are advocates of pain management in a variety of ways. In 2002 Christine Miaskowski, a dual member of ASPMN and APS, became the first nurse elected as President of APS. Today, ASPMN provides position statements regarding pain management, participates in the development of legislation related to pain, provides numerous continuing education events in pain management, and reports on pain-relieving strategies that are evidence-based and ethical. In 2002 ASPMN published its *Core Curriculum for Pain Management Nursing* (St. Marie) to foster the inclusion of pain management courses in nursing programs and to provide an inclusive framework for practicing nurses.

Since the 1960s, nurses have continued to be involved with and have an impact on the care of patients with pain (Johnson & Rice 1974; Kaufman et al. 1961; Larkins 1977; Lindemann 1975). They serve on committees and boards of nursing and medical organizations that focus on pain management. Nurses provide expert leadership for the development of guidelines for pain management in a variety of populations. APS has promoted universal awareness of pain by publishing guidelines on the management of cancer and acute pain with nursing involvement (Payne et al. 1987). The APS continues to seek interdisciplinary participation in updates of these guidelines (Ashburn et al. 2003; Max et al. 1998) and to develop pain management guidelines for specific pain syndromes, including sickle cell disease (Benjamin et al. 1999) and arthritis (Simon et al. 2002).

In 1992 the Agency for Healthcare Research and Quality (AHRQ), then the Agency for Health Care Policy and Research, established guidelines (reviewed by nurses) for the treatment of acute pain (Carr et al.). This was followed in 1994 (Jacox et al.) and 2000 (Welsh et al.) by guidelines for cancer pain. Several guidelines are now available on the AHRQ Web site (http://www.ahrq.gov/clinic/epcindex.htm).

The American Geriatrics Society revised *The Management of Chronic Pain in Older Persons* (1998) to *The Management of Persistent Pain in Older Persons* (2002) with the help of nurses on the Expert Panel and among the peer reviewers. In January 2001, the Joint Commission on Accreditation of Healthcare Organizations (JCAHO) implemented the pain standard that all JCAHO-approved agencies must meet. These events, as well as the proliferation of pain research, have contributed to the development of the theory that pain is not simply considered a symptom of disease, but is regarded as a co-morbid medical condition. This paradigm shift resulted in Congress designating the years 2001 through 2010 as the Decade of Pain Control and Research, with the objective of making pain more visible and more appropriately treated.

Characteristics of Specialty Practice

In accord with *Nursing's Social Policy Statement* (ANA 2003a), pain management nurses address societal issues of health and wellness by protecting, promoting, and restoring the health of patients with pain. They are aware that certain populations, including but not limited to neonates, children, adolescents, elders, the mentally challenged, patients with acute, neurological trauma, and those with previous or current substance abuse, are at risk for inadequate pain management. Pain management nurses strive to overcome patient, family, healthcare provider, healthcare agency, and legal barriers to effective pain management in these and other populations. They also recognize institutional and financial impediments to effective pain management and work to remove them. Pain management nurses collaborate with medical and nursing organizations to promote prevention of pain and optimal treatment of pain while discouraging abuse and diversion of opioids.

Pain management nursing continues to advance as a profession with a distinct body of knowledge that is evidence-based and ethically sound—based on *Code of Ethics for Nurses with Interpretive Statements* (ANA 2001). The scope of pain management nursing practice is guided by: federal and state laws and regulations, evidence-based clinical research, expert-based opinions, professional organizations, position statements and guidelines, standards of care, and the code of ethics.

Pain is the primary symptom that drives patients to seek medical attention. Universally, nurses in diverse settings encounter patients with various types and degrees of pain who are also developmentally different, including elders, adults, adolescents, children, infants, and neonates.

While the responsibilities of the role may vary from state to state and from practice setting to practice setting, the nurse whose specialty is pain management is expected to apply evidence-based knowledge, including but not limited to:

- functional neuroanatomy;
- nociceptive and neuropathic processes;
- psychosocial responses to pain;
- common situations, diseases, and syndromes associated with acute, chronic, and neuropathic pain;
- valid and reliable methods of pain assessment;
- evidence-based practice guidelines for pharmacologic and non-pharmacologic interventions for pain;
- methods for measuring, monitoring, evaluating, and documenting pain interventions and outcomes;
- and age-appropriate and culturally sensitive pain interventions.

Distinct levels of nursing practice relative to pain management have emerged as a result of this continued expansion of pain management knowledge (Pellino et al. 2002). In *Nursing's Social Policy Statement* (2003a), the American Nurses Association defined nursing as "the prevention of illness, the alleviation of suffering, and the protection, promotion, and restoration of health in the care of individuals, families, groups, communities, and populations." In 2003, in the revised position statement Pain Management and Control of Distressing Symptoms in Dying Patients, the ANA Board of Directors (2003b) stated, "When the restoration of health is no longer possible, the focus of nursing care is assuring a comfortable, dignified death and the highest possible quality of remaining life."… "The assessment and management of pain… must be based on an informed understanding of the individual patient's values and goals and his/her emotional, physical, and spiritual needs as well as on an understanding of the pathophysiology of the disease state and evidence-based palliative care practice" The statement goes on to endorse the responsibility of the licensed professional nurse in assessing and managing pain.

The American Society of Pain Management Nurses, in its blueprint for practice, *Core Curriculum for Pain Management Nursing* (St. Marie 2002), states, "The professional nurse uses a nursing model and framework to generate an individual plan of care based on the nursing process and the individual's response to illness, incorporating efforts and the individual's preferences for the safe management and relief of pain and suffering" (6). These and many other references and organizations, including JCAHO, provide policy statements and regulations that stipulate a standard of care in the assessment and management of pain for each licensed professional nurse regardless of general practice, specialty practice, or advanced practice designation. Evidence-based theoretical knowledge and competence in clinical practice is integrated into the nursing process, and in some cases the medical model, to promote acceptable clinical outcomes.

Roles and Specialty Practice

The roles of the registered nurse and of the advanced practice nurse are established by the profession and are described in the scope of nursing practice and scope of specialty nursing practice statements. Nursing practice is further defined by evidence-based and expert-based position statements, guidelines, standards of care, and state nurse practice acts, statutes, and regulations. Nurses then incorporate this knowledge into practice in the orderly and integrated process of assessment, planning, intervention, and evaluation of the individual patient in context to health and illness, considering internal and external variables within the patient's environment. As the licensed professional nurse becomes more proficient and acquires additional knowledge and certifications, practice evolves from novice to the expert and role model levels. This progression often includes additional educational preparation and recognition or licensure as an advanced practice registered nurse with an expanded scope of practice, including advanced diagnostic skills and prescriptive privileges.

The core of pain management nursing applies the processes of prevention, assessment, treatment, evaluation, and rehabilitation to the multidimensional and individualized aspects of pain. The pain management nurse provides direct patient care while facilitating and coordinating an individualized pain management plan through application of the nursing process and through personal knowledge of the patient. An effective pain management plan is derived from an understanding of the pathophysiology of pain and the influence of an individual's biopsychosocial needs on pain perception and response.

When implementing the nursing process, the pain management nurse assesses pain, plans pain management strategies, provides safe, individualized pain-relieving interventions, and evaluates the effectiveness or adverse effects of these interventions. As the patient's advocate who recognizes the importance of the patient's values, goals, and preferences, the pain management nurse uses effective communication skills and collaborates and coordinates the pain plan of care with the patient/family, physician, and other healthcare providers.

Pain management nursing addresses the multidimensional aspects of pain while promoting an interdisciplinary approach to provide a multimodal plan of care. The pain management nurse participates in interdisciplinary patient care conferences, provides patient/family education, counseling, and discharge planning, and facilitates rehabilitative, palliative, and end-of-life pain management. Furthermore, the pain management nurse assists in the development of pain management policies, participates in research data collection, teaches ancillary personnel specific and appropriate aspects of pain management, mentors or serves as a resource for nurses with limited pain management knowledge, and continually stays up to date by reviewing current literature, attending conferences, and initiating or participating in collegial dialogue (St. Marie 2002).

Advanced Practice Registered Nurses

The Advanced Practice Registered Nurse (APRN) who specializes in pain management is most often a Clinical Nurse Specialist (CNS) or a Nurse Practitioner (NP). The CNS role has required Master's preparation since its inception, while the American Nurses Association has required NP preparation at the Master's level since 1992. The APRN makes independent and collaborative pain management decisions (American Academy of Nurse Practitioners 2002).

The CNS "receives components of pain management theory and clinical practice within the auspices of symptom management for their specialty population" (St. Marie 2002, 532). The CNS in pain management practices primarily in the acute inpatient setting. The pain management CNS is a clinical expert who may provide direct patient care, but is more often involved in:

- designing, implementing, and evaluating pain programs;
- serving as a leader, consultant, and change agent in pain management;
- leading multidisciplinary pain management teams;
- providing staff education in pain management;
- participating in pain quality improvement activities;
- identifying clinical pain management problems;
- initiating clinical research of pain management problems;
- and serving as a resource for nurses and other clinicians, consulting on patients with complex pain problems.

The CNS may also function as an administrative leader—ensuring optimal pain personnel coverage, being accountable for reimbursement of pain interventions, and evaluating pain-relieving products (St. Marie 2002).

The NP in pain management functions both interdependently and independently in assessing and managing both medical and nursing problems related to pain, primarily in patients in the acute care, outpatient, or clinic settings. Patients with pain are of all ages: neonates, infants, children, adolescents, adults, and elders. Long-term care facilities, home health, hospices, and other settings value the services of the nurse practitioner specializing in pain management.

The pain management NP focuses on preventing pain and discouraging patients from engaging in pain-provoking activities, reflective of the American Academy of Nurse Practitioners *Nurse Practitioner as an Advanced Practice Nurse Role Position Statement* (2002): "their practice emphasizes health promotion and maintenance, disease prevention, and the diagnosis and management of acute and chronic diseases." Pain management NPs collaborate with other disciplines and specialists in developing a pain management plan for patients with transient/acute and persistent/chronic pain syndromes when pain prevention strategies fail.

Pain management NPs recognize "the symptom of pain as a fundamental part of the differential diagnosis process" (St. Marie 2002, 541). However, they also understand that the experience of pain is complex and multi-dimensional, often involving the whole person. Thus, NPs conduct comprehensive pain assessments that incorporate a history of the pain, including previously tried pain-relieving interventions (pharmacological, herbal, and over-the-counter drugs); current co-morbid medical conditions; a physical examination; and psychological, social, emotional, and spiritual assessments. The pain management NP orders diagnostic tests to aid in the differential diagnosis of the cause of the pain, which will determine treatment.

Pain management NPs set pain management goals with the patient or family, develop and initiate a comprehensive pain treatment plan, educate the patient or family regarding the pain and pain plan, and evaluate the effectiveness of the pain plan in relieving the patient's pain or restoring patient function and quality of life. Pain management NPs' practices are regulated by the NPs' state of licensure, which determines the level of independent practice and the authority to prescribe controlled and non-controlled medications. Practice varies from independent to variable collaborative agreements to direct supervision.

Specialty Certification

ASPMN initially developed nursing practice standards with *Standards of Clinical Nursing Practice for Pain Management* (1996) and *Standards of Clinical Practice for the Specialty of Pain Management Nursing* (1998). In 2002 ASPMN set forth a blueprint for current pain management theory and practice in nursing with *Curriculum for Pain Management Nursing* (St. Marie). The American Nurses Credentialing Center (ANCC) partnered with ASPMN to develop a certification process for pain management based on this blueprint, in which certification is conferred after a combination of examination and clinical practice. The completion of the core curriculum provided a basis to operationalize the standards of pain management nursing detailed on the following pages.

Trends and Issues

Nursing as a profession has the responsibility to advocate for adequate and appropriate pain control for all patients. Pain management nurses should be prepared to lobby for the following:

- improved pain competency in nurses;
- certification and advanced degrees in pain management;
- refinement and clarification of pain standards;
- enhanced use of non-pharmacological strategies for pain management that are evidence-based;
- development of position papers and guidelines for pain management in special populations;
- improved pain management in populations at highest risk for undertreatment of pain;
- increased patient pain education;
- better funding for well controlled, nurse-conducted pain research;
- more active roles in legislation and government relations;
- and expansion of the role of the nurse as the primary pain manager (Pasero 2003).

As knowledge of pain management continues to grow, newer physical, cognitive-behavioral, and interventional modalities will appear; novel pharmaceuticals based on basic research of pain pathophysiology will be developed; and new technologically advanced modalities will emerge. Environments in which nurses care for patients with pain will change. The culture of patients with pain will be more diverse.

Evidence-based practice derived from a sound theoretical framework will prepare pain management nurses to critically analyze objective data and integrate it with patients' subjective pain experience. They will be prepared to communicate effectively with a variety of healthcare providers, legislators, and the media on pain issues. Through active participation in civic activities, including membership in and support of professional organizations, pain management nurses will continue to influence the direction of pain management.

Pain management nurses must be flexible and dynamic, proactive instead of reactive; they must lead efforts to influence the future of pain management. The profession of nursing must use caution in accepting current or new practices in pain management, and ensure that these practices are based on credible research and improved patient outcomes.

STANDARDS OF PAIN MANAGEMENT NURSING PRACTICE

STANDARDS OF PRACTICE

STANDARD 1. ASSESSMENT

The registered nurse collects comprehensive data pertinent to the pain problem.

Measurement Criteria:

The registered nurse:

- Collects data and identifies patterns and the impact of pain in a systematic and ongoing process.
- Involves the patient, family, and other healthcare providers, as appropriate, in comprehensive data collection.
- Determines the priority of data collection activities by the patient's immediate condition or anticipated needs.
- Uses appropriate evidence-based pain assessment tools and techniques that are developmentally, cognitively, and culturally sensitive.
- Uses analytical models and problem-solving tools.
- Documents relevant data that facilitates retrieval, reassessment, and follow up.
- Synthesizes available data, information, and knowledge relevant to the patient in pain.

Additional Measurement Criterion for the Advanced Practice Registered Nurse:
The advanced practice registered nurse:

- Initiates and interprets diagnostic tests and procedures relevant to the patient's current pain status.

STANDARD 2. DIAGNOSIS

The registered nurse analyzes the assessment data to determine pain diagnoses or problems.

Measurement Criteria:

The registered nurse:

- Derives the diagnoses or problems based on assessment data.
- Validates the diagnoses or problems with the patient, family, and other healthcare providers when possible and appropriate.
- Prioritizes pain-related diagnoses or problems based on special needs of the patient.
- Documents diagnoses or problems in a manner that facilitates the determination of the expected outcomes and plan.

Additional Measurement Criteria for the Advanced Practice Registered Nurse:

The advanced practice registered nurse:

- Systematically compares and contrasts complex clinical findings with normal and abnormal variations and developmental events in formulating an individual diagnosis.
- Uses complex data and information obtained during interview, physical examination, and diagnostic procedures in formulating pain diagnoses.
- Assists nursing staff in developing and maintaining competency in the diagnostic processes related to pain management.

STANDARD 3. OUTCOMES IDENTIFICATION

The registered nurse identifies expected pain management outcomes for a plan individualized to the patient with pain.

Measurement Criteria:

The registered nurse:

- Involves the patient, family, and other healthcare providers in formulating mutually expected outcomes when possible and appropriate.
- Derives culturally appropriate expected outcomes from the diagnoses.
- Considers associated risks, benefits, costs, current scientific evidence, and clinical expertise when formulating expected outcomes of pain management strategies.
- Defines expected outcomes in terms of the patient, patient values, ethical considerations, environment, or situation with such consideration as associated risks, benefits, costs, and current scientific evidence.
- Includes a time estimate for attainment of expected outcomes.
- Develops expected outcomes that provide direction for continuity of care.
- Modifies expected outcomes based on changes in the status of the patient or evaluation of the situation.
- Documents expected outcomes as measurable goals.

Additional Measurement Criteria for the Advanced Practice Registered Nurse:

The advanced practice registered nurse:

- Identifies expected outcomes that incorporate scientific evidence and are achievable through implementation of evidence-based practices.
- Identifies expected outcomes that incorporate cost and clinical effectiveness, patient satisfaction, and continuity and consistency among providers.
- Supports the use of clinical guidelines linked to positive patient outcomes.

Standard 4. Planning

The registered nurse develops a pain management plan that prescribes strategies and alternatives to attain expected outcomes.

Measurement Criteria:

The registered nurse:

- Develops an individualized pain management plan, considering patient characteristics or the situation (e.g. age- and culture-appropriate, environmentally sensitive).
- Develops the pain management plan in conjunction with the patient, family, and others as appropriate.
- Includes strategies within the pain management plan that address each of the identified diagnoses or issues, which may include strategies for promotion and restoration of health and prevention of pain-producing illness, injury, or disease.
- Provides for continuity with the pain management plan.
- Incorporates an implementation pathway or timeline within the pain management plan.
- Establishes pain management plan priorities with the patient, family, and others as appropriate.
- Uses the pain management plan to provide direction to other members of the healthcare team.
- Defines the pain management plan to reflect current statutes, rules, regulations, and standards.
- Integrates current trends and research affecting pain management in the planning process.
- Considers the economic impact of the pain management plan.
- Uses standardized language or recognized terminology to document the pain management plan.

Additional Measurement Criteria for the Advanced Practice Registered Nurse:

The advanced practice registered nurse:

- Identifies assessment, diagnostic strategies, and therapeutic interventions within the pain management plan that reflect current evidence, including data, research, literature, and expert clinical knowledge.
- Selects or designs pain-relieving strategies to meet the multifaceted needs of patients with complex pain syndromes.
- Includes the synthesis of patient's values and beliefs regarding nursing and medical therapies with the pain management plan.

STANDARD 5. IMPLEMENTATION

The registered nurse implements the identified pain management plan.

Measurement Criteria:

The registered nurse:

- Implements the pain management plan in a safe and timely manner.
- Documents implementation and any modifications, including changes or omissions, of the identified pain management plan
- Uses evidence-based interventions and treatments specific to the diagnosis of pain.
- Uses community resources and systems to implement the pain management plan.
- Collaborates with nursing colleagues and others to implement the pain management plan.

Additional Measurement Criteria for the Advanced Practice Registered Nurse:

The advanced practice registered nurse:

- Facilitates utilization of systems and community resources to implement the pain management plan.
- Supports collaboration with nursing colleagues and other disciplines to implement the pain management plan.
- Incorporates new knowledge and strategies to initiate change in nursing pain care practices if desired outcomes are not achieved.

STANDARD 5A. COORDINATION OF CARE

The registered nurse coordinates the pain management plan.

Measurement Criteria:

The registered nurse:

- Coordinates implementation of the pain management plan.
- Documents coordination of care.

Additional Measurement Criteria for the Advanced Practice Registered Nurse:

The advanced practice registered nurse:

- Provides leadership in the coordination of interdisciplinary health care for integrated delivery of the individualized pain management plan.
- Synthesizes data and information to prescribe necessary system and community support measures, including environmental modifications.
- Coordinates system and community resources that enhance delivery of effective pain management across systems.

STANDARD 5B. HEALTH TEACHING AND HEALTH PROMOTION

The registered nurse employs strategies to promote, maintain, and restore pain-relieving behaviors.

Measurement Criteria:

The registered nurse:

- Provides health teaching on such topics as pain prevention lifestyles, pain-reducing behaviors, developmental needs, activities of daily living, and self-care within the context of the patient's co-morbid features.

- Uses health promotion and health teaching methods appropriate to the situation and the patient's developmental needs, readiness, ability to learn, language preference, and culture.

- Seeks opportunities for feedback and evaluation of the effectiveness of pain-relieving strategies used.

Additional Measurement Criteria for the Advanced Practice Registered Nurse:

The advanced practice registered nurse:

- Synthesizes empirical evidence on risk behaviors, learning theories, behavioral change theories, motivational theories, epidemiology, and other related theories and frameworks when designing health information and patient education related to pain management.

- Designs appropriate pain management education appropriate to the patient's developmental level, learning needs, readiness to learn, and cultural values and beliefs.

- Evaluates pain information resources, such as the Internet, within the area of practice for accuracy, readability, and comprehensibility to help patients access quality pain management information.

STANDARD 5C. CONSULTATION

The advanced practice registered nurse provides consultation to influence the identified pain management plan, enhance the abilities of others, and effect change.

Additional Measurement Criteria for the Advanced Practice Registered Nurse: The advanced practice registered nurse:

- Synthesizes data, information, theoretical frameworks, and evidence on pain management when providing consultation.

- Facilitates the effectiveness of a consultation by involving the patient and other stakeholders in the pain management decision-making process and negotiating role responsibilities.

- Communicates consultation recommendations that influence the pain management plan, facilitate understanding by involved stakeholders, enhance the work of others, and effect change.

Standards of Professional Performance

Standard 7. Quality of Practice

The registered nurse systematically evaluates the quality and effectiveness of pain management practice.

Measurement Criteria:

The registered nurse:

- Demonstrates quality by documenting the application of the nursing process in a responsible, accountable, and ethical manner.
- Uses results of quality improvement activities to initiate changes in nursing pain practice and in the healthcare delivery system.
- Uses creativity and innovation in nursing practice to improve pain management.
- Incorporates new knowledge to initiate changes in pain nursing practice if desired outcomes are not achieved.
- Participates in quality improvement activities. Such activities may include:
  - Identifying aspects of pain practice important for quality monitoring.
  - Using indicators developed to monitor quality and effectiveness of pain nursing practice.
  - Collecting data to monitor quality and effectiveness of pain interventions.
  - Analyzing pain management quality data to identify opportunities for improving pain management practice.
  - Formulating recommendations to improve pain management nursing practice or outcomes.
  - Implementing pain-relieving activities to enhance the quality of pain management nursing practice.
  - Developing, implementing, and evaluating policies, procedures, and guidelines to improve the quality of nursing pain management.
  - Participating on interdisciplinary teams to evaluate clinical outcomes of pain management or pain management health services.

- Participating in efforts to minimize costs and unnecessary duplication of pain management services.
- Analyzing factors related to safety, satisfaction, effectiveness, and cost–benefit options related to pain management.
- Analyzing organizational systems for barriers to optimal pain management.
- Implementing processes to remove or decrease barriers to optimal pain management.

Additional Measurement Criteria for the Advanced Practice Registered Nurse:

The advanced practice registered nurse:

- Obtains and maintains professional certification in pain management.
- Designs quality improvement initiatives related to pain management.
- Initiates evaluation of the need for change to optimize pain management.
- Evaluates the practice environment and the quality of pain nursing care delivered in relation to existing evidence, identifying opportunities for research.

STANDARD 8. EDUCATION

The registered nurse attains knowledge and competency that reflects current pain management nursing practice.

Measurement Criteria:

The registered nurse:

- Participates in ongoing pain management education related to appropriate knowledge bases and professional issues.
- Demonstrates a commitment to lifelong learning through self-reflection and inquiry to identify pain management learning needs.
- Seeks experiences that reflect current evidence-based pain management practice to maintain skills and competence in the clinical practice of pain management or role performance.
- Acquires knowledge and skills appropriate to the pain management specialty area, practice setting, role, or situation.
- Maintains professional records that provide evidence of competency and lifelong learning related to pain management.
- Seeks experiences and formal and independent learning activities to maintain and develop pain management clinical and professional skills and knowledge.

Additional Measurement Criterion for the Advanced Practice Registered Nurse:

The advanced practice registered nurse:

- Uses current healthcare research findings and other evidence to expand clinical knowledge, enhance role performance, and increase knowledge of pain management.

STANDARD 9. PROFESSIONAL PRACTICE EVALUATION

The registered nurse evaluates their own nursing practice in relation to professional pain practice standards and guidelines, relevant statutes, rules, and regulations.

Measurement Criteria:

The registered nurse's practice reflects the application of knowledge of current pain practice standards, guidelines, statutes, rules, and regulations.

The registered nurse:

- Provides age-appropriate pain management in a culturally and ethnically sensitive manner.
- Engages in self-evaluation of practice on a regular basis, identifying areas of strengths as well as areas in which professional development would be beneficial.
- Obtains informal feedback regarding their own practice from patients, peers, professional colleagues, and others.
- Participates in systematic peer review as appropriate.
- Takes action to achieve goals identified during the evaluation process.
- Provides rationales for pain practice beliefs, decisions, and actions as part of the informal and formal evaluation processes.

Additional Measurement Criteria for the Advanced Practice Registered Nurse:

The advanced practice registered nurse:

- Engages in a formal process seeking feedback regarding their own pain management practice from patients, peers, professional colleagues, and others.

STANDARD 10. COLLEGIALITY

The registered nurse interacts with, and contributes to the professional development of, peers and colleagues.

Measurement Criteria:

The registered nurse:

- Shares pain management knowledge and skills with peers and colleagues as evidenced by such activities as patient care conferences or presentations at formal or informal meetings.

- Provides peers with constructive feedback regarding their pain management practice or role performance.

- Interacts with peers and colleagues to enhance the nurse's own professional pain management practice or role performance.

- Maintains compassionate and caring relationships with peers and colleagues.

- Contributes to an environment that is conducive to the pain management education of healthcare providers.

- Contributes to a supportive and healthy work environment.

Additional Measurement Criteria for the Advanced Practice Registered Nurse:

The advance practice registered nurse:

- Models expert pain management practice to interdisciplinary team members and healthcare consumers.

- Mentors other registered nurses and colleagues as appropriate.

- Participates with interdisciplinary teams who contribute to role development and advanced nursing practice and health care.

Standard 11. Collaboration

The registered nurse collaborates with patient, family, and others in the conduct of pain management nursing practice.

Measurement Criteria:

The registered nurse:

- Communicates with patient, family, and healthcare providers regarding the pain management plan and the nurse's role in the provision of that plan.

- Collaborates in creating a documented plan, focused on pain relief outcomes and decisions related to care and delivery of pain-relieving strategies, that demonstrates communication with patients, families, and others.

- Partners with others to effect change and to generate positive pain management outcomes through knowledge of the patient or situation.

- Documents referrals, including provisions for continuity of pain management.

Additional Measurement Criteria for the Advanced Practice Registered Nurse:

The advanced practice registered nurse:

- Partners with other disciplines to enhance patient care through interdisciplinary activities, such as education, consultation, management, technological development, or research opportunities.

- Facilitates an interdisciplinary process with other members of the healthcare team.

- Documents plan of care communications, rationales for changes in the plan of care, and collaborative discussions to improve pain management.

STANDARD 12. ETHICS

The registered nurse integrates ethical provisions to guide pain management practices.

Measurement Criteria:

The registered nurse:

- Uses *Code of Ethics for Nurses with Interpretive Statements* (ANA 2001) to guide practice.
- Delivers pain management in a manner that preserves and protects patient autonomy, dignity, and rights.
- Maintains patient confidentiality within legal and regulatory parameters.
- Serves as a patient advocate and helps patients experiencing pain to develop skills for self-advocacy.
- Maintains a therapeutic and professional nurse–patient relationship within appropriate professional boundaries.
- Demonstrates a commitment to practicing self-care, managing stress, and connecting with self and others.
- Contributes to resolving ethical issues of patients, colleagues, or systems, as evidenced in such activities as participating on ethics committees.
- Reports illegal, incompetent, or impaired pain management practices.

Additional Measurement Criteria for the Advanced Practice Registered Nurse:

The advanced practice registered nurse:

- Informs the patient of the risks, benefits, and outcomes of the pain management plan.
- Participates in interdisciplinary teams that address ethical risks, benefits, and outcomes of the pain management plan.

STANDARD 13. RESEARCH

The registered nurse integrates pain research findings into clinical practice.

Measurement Criteria:

The registered nurse:

- Uses the best available evidence, including research findings, to guide pain practice decisions.
- Actively participates in research activities at various levels appropriate to the nurse's level of education and position. Such activities may include:
  - Identifying clinical pain management problems specific to nursing research.
  - Participating in data collection (e.g. surveys, pilot projects, formal studies).
  - Participating in a formal committee or program.
  - Sharing pain research activities and findings with peers and others.
  - Conducting research.
  - Using research findings in the development of policies, procedures, and standards of practice in pain management.
  - Incorporating research as a basis for learning.

Additional Measurement Criteria for the Advanced Practice Registered Nurse:

The advanced practice registered nurse:

- Contributes to pain management nursing knowledge by conducting or synthesizing research that discovers, examines, and evaluates knowledge, theories, criteria, and creative approaches to improving pain management.
- Formally disseminates research findings through activities such as presentations, publications, consultation, and journal clubs.

STANDARD 14. RESOURCE UTILIZATION

The registered nurse considers factors related to safety, effectiveness, cost, and impact on practice in the planning and delivery of pain management.

Measurement Criteria:

The registered nurse:

- Evaluates factors such as safety, effectiveness, availability, cost and benefits, efficiencies, and impact on practice when choosing pain management options that would result in the same expected outcome.

- Assists the patient and family in identifying and securing appropriate and available services to address pain-related needs.

- Assigns or delegates pain-relieving tasks, based on needs and condition of the patient, potential for harm, stability of the patient's condition, complexity of the task, and predictability of the outcome.

- Assists the patient and family in becoming informed consumers about the options, cost, risks, and benefits of pain management strategies.

Additional Measurement Criteria for the Advanced Practice Registered Nurse:

The advanced practice registered nurse:

- Uses organizational and community resources to formulate multidisciplinary or interdisciplinary pain management plans.

- Develops innovative solutions for pain management problems that address effective resource utilization and maintenance of quality.

- Develops evaluation strategies to demonstrate cost effectiveness, cost benefit, and efficiency factors associated with nursing pain management.

STANDARD 15. LEADERSHIP

The registered nurse provides leadership in professional pain management.

Measurement Criteria:

The registered nurse:

- Works as a team player and team builder.
- Works to create and maintain healthy work environments in local, regional, national, or international pain management communities.
- Displays the ability to define a clear vision, the associated goals, and a pain management plan to implement and measure progress.
- Demonstrates a commitment to continuous, lifelong learning for self and others.
- Teaches others to succeed by mentoring and other strategies.
- Exhibits creativity and flexibility through times of change.
- Demonstrates energy, excitement, and passion for quality pain management.
- Willingly accepts mistakes by self and others, thereby creating a culture in which risk-taking is not only safe, but expected.
- Inspires loyalty by valuing people as the most precious asset in an organization.
- Directs the coordination of care across settings and among caregivers, including oversight of licensed and unlicensed personnel in any assigned or delegated tasks.
- Serves in key roles in the work setting by participating on committees, councils, and administrative teams.
- Promotes advancement of the profession through participation in professional organizations.

Additional Measurement Criteria for the Advanced Practice Registered Nurse:

The advanced practice registered nurse:

- Works to influence decision-making bodies to improve pain management.
- Provides direction to enhance the effectiveness of the healthcare team.
- Initiates and revises pain management protocols or guidelines to reflect evidence-based pain management practice, to reflect accepted changes in pain management, or to address emerging pain management problems.
- Promotes communication of information and advancement of the profession through writing, publishing, and presentation for professional or lay audiences.
- Designs innovations to effect change in practice and improve health outcomes.

GLOSSARY

Client. The recipient of care: an individual, family, group, or community. When the client is an individual, the focus is on the health state, problems, or needs of that person. When the client is a family or group, the focus is on the health state of the unit as a whole or the effects of the individual's health state on the other members of the unit. When the client is a community, the focus is on the personal and environmental health states and the health risks of population groups. Nursing actions for clients may be directed toward disease, illness, or injury prevention, health restoration, or health maintenance.

Criteria. Relevant, measurable indicators of the standards of clinical nursing practice.

Healthcare team. A set of individuals with special expertise who provide healthcare services or assistance to clients. They may include nurses, physicians, psychologists, social workers, nutritionists/dieticians, and various therapists. Healthcare providers also may include service organizations and vendors. A team is comprised of a number of persons associated together in work or activity.

Holism (holistic). A view of the universe that focuses on its interconnected patterns and processes that combine to form a whole instead of a collection of fragmented parts. *Holistic nursing* has as its goal the health and healing of the whole person, based on the entwined assumptions that the parts of a patient are intimately interconnected and that physical, mental, social, and spiritual factors need to be included in any interventions. Holism involves understanding the individual as an integrated whole who interacts with and is acted upon by both internal and external environments.

Interdisciplinary. Reliant on the overlapping skills and knowledge of each team member and discipline, resulting in synergistic effects where outcomes are enhanced and more comprehensive than the simple aggregation of any team member's individual efforts.

Multidisciplinary. Relating to, or using a combination of, several disciplines for a common purpose. A multidisciplinary team is a unit composed of individuals with varied and specialized expertise who coordinate their activities to provide diagnostic and therapeutic services to clients with an actual or potential diagnosis. The team engages in collaborative endeavors using the combined skills and expertise of team members. The client is a member of the team whenever possible and appropriate.

Role. A function, especially the characteristic and expected social behavior of an individual in relationship to a group.

Standard. An authoritative statement enunciated and promulgated by the profession, by which the quality of practice, service, or education can be judged.

REFERENCES

American Academy of Nurse Practitioners, 2002. *Nurse practitioner as an advanced practice nurse role.* Position Statement. Office of Health Policy. Washington, DC: AANP.

American Geriatric Society (1998). The management of persistent pain in older persons. (2002). *Journal of the American Geriatrics Society* 50 (6): S205-S224.

American Nurses Association. 1987. *Scope of nursing practice.* Kansas City, MO: ANA.

———. 2001. *Code of ethics for nurses with interpretive statements.* Washington, DC: American Nurses Publishing.

———. 2003a. *Nursing's social policy statement, 2nd edition.* Washington, DC: nursesbooks.org.

———. 2003b. *Pain management and control of distressing symptoms in dying patients.* Position Statement. Washington, DC: ANA.

———. 2004. *Nursing: Scope and standards of practice.* Washington, DC: nursesbooks.org.

American Society of Pain Management Nurses. 1996. *Standards of clinical nursing practice for pain management.* Pensacola, FL: ASPMN.

———. 1997. *Certification philosophy.* (November 23). Pensacola, FL: ASPMN.

———. 1998. *Standards of clinical nursing practice for the specialty of pain management nursing.* Pensacola, FL: ASPMN.

Ashburn, M., D. Carr, A. Lipman, & C. Rubingh. 2003. *American Pain Society guidelines. Principles of analgesic use in the treatment of acute pain and cancer pain,* 5th ed. Glenview, IL: APS.

Benjamin, L., C. Dampier, A. Jacox, V. Odesina, D. Phoenix, B. Shapiro, M. Strafford, & M. Treadwell. 1999. *American Pain Society guideline: Guideline for the management of acute and chronic pain in sickle-cell disease.* Glenview, IL: APS.

Carr, D., A. Jacox, C. Chapman, B. Ferrell, H. Fields, G. Heidrich, N. Hester, C. Hill, A. Lipman, C. McGarvey, C. Miaskowski, D. Mulder, R. Payne, N. Schecter, B. Shapiro, R. Smith, C. Tsou, & L. Vecchiarelli. 1992. *Clinical practice guideline: Acute pain management: Operative or medical procedures and trauma.* Pub. No. 92-0032. Rockville, MD: Agency for Health Care Policy and Research.

Crowley, D. 1962. *Pain and its alleviation*. Los Angeles: University of California at Los Angeles School of Nursing.

Greipp, M.E. 1992. Undermedication for pain: An ethical model. *Advances in Nursing Science* 15 (1): 44–53 (PMID# 1519910).

International Association for the Study of Pain. 1974. *Articles of incorporation and bylaws*. University of Washington School of Medicine, Department of Anesthesia. Seattle, WA: IASP.

Jacox, A. 1977. *Pain: A source book for nurses and other health professionals*. Boston: Little, Brown, and Company.

Jacox, A., & M. Steward. 1978. *Psychosocial contingencies of the pain experience*. Iowa City: University of Iowa.

Jacox, A., D. Carr, R. Payne, C. Berde, W. Briebart, J. Cain, C. Chapman, C. Cleeland, B. Ferrell, R. Finley, N. Hester, C. Hill, W. Leak, A. Lipman, C. Logan, C. McGarvey, C. Miaskowski, D. Mulder, J. Paice, B. Shapiro, E. Silberstein, R. Smith, J. Stover, C. Tsou, L. Vecchiarelli, & D. Weissman. 1994. *Clinical practice guideline: Management of cancer pain*. Pub. No. 94-0592. Rockville, MD: Agency for Health Care Policy and Research.

Johnson, J.E., & V.H. Rice. 1974. Sensory and distress components of pain: Implications for the study of clinical pain. *Nursing Research* 23 (May–June): 203–209.

Joint Commission on Accreditation of Healthcare Organizations (JACHO). 2000–2004. *Comprehensive accreditation manual for hospitals: The official handbook*. (Annual publication). Oak Brook Terrace, IL: JCAHO.

Kaufman, M., & D. Brown. 1961. Pain wears many faces. *American Journal of Nursing* LXI (January): 48–51.

Larkins, F.R. 1977. The influences of one patient's culture on pain response. *Nursing Clinics of North America* 12 (December): 663–668.

Lindemann, C.A. 1975. Priorities in clinical nursing research. *Nursing Outlook* 23 (November): 693–698.

Max, M., R. Payne, T. Edwards, A. Sunshine, & C. Inturrisi. 1998. *American Pain Society guideline: Principles of analgesic use in the treatment of acute pain and cancer pain*, 4th ed. Glenview, IL: APS.

McCaffery, M. 1968. *Nursing practice theories related to cognition, bodily pain, and man–environment interactions*. Los Angeles: University of California.

———. 1972. *Nursing management of the patient with pain*. Philadelphia: J.B. Lippincott Company.

————. 1979. *Nursing management of the patient with pain,* 2nd ed. Philadelphia: J.B. Lippincott Company.

McCaffery, M., & A. Beebe. 1989. *Pain: Clinical manual for nursing practice.* St. Louis: C.V. Mosby.

McCaffery, M., & C. Pasero. 1999. *Pain: Clinical manual,* 2nd ed. St. Louis: C.V. Mosby.

Melzack, R., & P.D. Wall. 1965. Pain and mechanisms: A new theory. *Science* 150:971–979.

————. 1983. *The Challenge of pain.* New York: Basic Books.

Merskey, H. (chairman). 1979. Pain terms: A list with definitions and notes on usage. *Pain* 6:249–252.

Pasero, C. 2003. *Standing the test of time: The nurse as primary pain manager.* Presentation at ASPMN National Convention, Kansas City, MO.

Payne, R., M. Max, C. Inturrisi, A. Rogers, A. Miser, S. Perry, and R. Kanner. 1987. *American Pain Society guideline: Principles of analgesic use in the treatment of acute pain and cancer pain. 3rd edition.* Skokie, IL: APS.

Pellino, T., J. Willens, R. Polomano, & M. Heye. 2002. The American Society of Pain Management Nurses practice analysis: Role delineation study. *Pain Management Nursing* 3 (1): 2–15.

Research! America. 2003. Public opinion polls: Pain. Alexandria, VA: *Research! America.* http://www.researchamerica.org/polldata/pain.html. Accessed February 25, 2005.

Rey, R. 1993. *The history of pain.* Cambridge, MA: Harvard University Press.

Rogers, A. 1967. Pain and the cancer patient. *Nursing Clinics of North America* 2: 671–682.

Simon, L., A. Lipman, A. Jacox, M. Caudill-Slosberg, L. Gill, F. Keefe, K. Kerr, M. Minor, D. Sherry, A. Vallerand, & S. Vasudevan, & C. Spengler. 1999. *American Pain Society guideline: Principles of analgesic use in the treatment of acute pain and cancer pain. 4th edition* Skokie, IL: APS.

Simon, L., A. Lipman, M. Caudill-Slosberg, L. Gill, F. Keefe, K. Kerr, M. Minor, D. Sherry, A. Vallerand, S. Vasudevan, and C. Spengler. 2002. *American Pain Society guideline for the management of pain in osteoarthritis, rheumatoid arthritis, and juvenile chronic arthritis.* Glenview, IL: APS.

St. Marie, B., ed. 2002. *Core curriculum for pain management nursing.* Philadelphia: W.B. Saunders.

Welsh, J., K. Copp, J. Dunne, B. Dymock, M. Emslie, M. Fallon, S. Fife, A. Harnett, J. Hockley, A. Hutcheon, B. Macrae, J. McElholm, D. Millar, S. Roche, F. Smith, M. Stevenson, J. Urie, & I. Wallace. 2000. *Control of pain in patients with cancer. A national clinical guideline.* Pub. No. 44. Edinburgh, Scotland: Agency for Healthcare Research and Quality.

World Health Organization. 1990. *Cancer pain relief and palliative care.* Albany, NY: WHO.

Index

C

Cancer pain, *vii*, 2, 3
   See also Pain
Care recipient. *See* Patient
   Care standards. *See* Standards
     of practice
   Case management. *See*
     Coordination of care
Certification and credentialing,
   1, 5, 7, 8
   education and, *vii*
   leadership and, 32
   quality of practice and, 24
Chronic pain, *v*, 3, 4, 7
   See also Pain
City of Hope, 1
Client (defined), 35
   See also Patient
Clinical Nurse Specialist (CNS), 6
Clinical settings. *See* Practice settings
Code of Ethics for Nurses with
   Interpretive Statements, vi, 3, 29
   See also Ethics
Collaboration, 3, 5
   diagnosis and, 12
   implementation and, 16
   leadership and, 32
   Nurse Practitioner and, 7
   standard of professional
     performance, 28
   See also Healthcare providers;
     Interdisciplinary health care
Collegiality, 6
   Clinical Nurse Specialist and, 6
   collaboration and, 28
   diagnosis and, 12
   ethics and, 29
   leadership and, 2, 32
   professional practice evaluation
     and, 26

research and, 2, 30
   standard of professional
     performance, 27
Communication, 5, 8, 9
   collaboration and, 28
   consultation and, 19
   ethics and, 29
   evaluation and, 21
   leadership and, 33
   research and, 30
Community health, 4, 9
   coordination of care and, 17
   implementation and, 16
   resource utilization and, 31
Competence assessment. *See*
  Certification and credentialing
Confidentiality, 29
   See also Ethics
Consultation, 6
   collaboration and, 28
   research and, 30
   standard of practice, 19
Continuity of care
   collaboration and, 28
   outcomes identification and, 13
   planning and, 14
Coordination of care, 5
   leadership and, 32
   standard of practice, 17
   See also Interdisciplinary
     health care
Core Curriculum for Pain Management
   Nursing, v–vi, vii, 2, 4, 8
Cost control, 3
   planning and, 14
   prescriptive authority and, 20
   quality of practice and, 24
   resource utilization and, 31
Cost-effectiveness. *See* Cost control
Credentialing. *See* Certification and
   credentialing

professional practice
  evaluation, 26
quality of practice, 23–24
research, 30
resource utilization, 31
roles, *vi*
See also Advanced practice pain
  management nursing; Pain
  management nursing
Guidelines
  development, *vi, vi,* 2–3, 4, 8
  leadership and, 33
  nursing roles, 5
  outcomes identification and, 13
  professional practice
    evaluation and, 26
  quality of practice and, 23

H
Health teaching and health
  promotion, 3, 4
  Nurse Practitioner and, 7
  planning and, 14
  standard of practice, 18
Healthcare policy
  evaluation and, 21
  pain management nursing
    and, 5, 6, 8, 9
  quality of practice and, 23
  research and, 30
Healthcare providers, 3
  assessment and, 11
  collaboration and, 5, 9, 28
  collegiality and, 27
  diagnosis and, 12
  evaluation and, 21
  leadership and, 32
  outcomes identification and, 13
  planning and, 14
  quality of practice and, 23
  See also Collaboration;
    Interdisciplinary health care

Healthcare team (defined), 35
  See also Collaboration;
    Interdisciplinary health care
Holistic practice, 7
  defined, 35
Human resources. *See* Professional
  development

I
Implementation
  evaluation and, 21
  planning and, 14
  standard of practice, 16–20
Information. *See* Data collection
Interdisciplinary health care, *vi,* 6
  collaboration and, 28
  Clinical Nurse Specialist and, 6
  collegiality and, 27
  coordination of care and, 17
  defined, 35
  ethics and, 29
  implementation and, 16
  leadership and, 32, 33
  quality of practice and, 23
  research and, 2
  resource utilization and, 31
  See also Collaboration;
    Healthcare providers
International Association for the
  Study of Pain (IASP), *v,* 1
Internet, 18
Interventions, 4, 5
  assessment and, 11
  evaluation and, 21
  planning and, 15

J
Joint Commission on Accreditation
  of Healthcare Organizations
  (JCAHO), *vi,* 3, 5

body of knowledge, 3
certification, 1, 5, 7, 8
characteristics, 3–5
Clinical Nurse Specialist, 6
cultural competence, *vi*
defined, 1
ethics, *vi*
generalist practice, 5–6
healthcare providers and, 3
history, 1–3
levels of practice, 4
Nurse Practitioner, 7
research, *v, vi,* 1–3, 6, 8, 9
roles, *vii*
scope of practice, 1–9
standards of practice, 11–21
standards of professional
    performance, 23–33
trends, 8–9
See also Advanced practice pain
    management nursing;
    Generalist pain management
    nursing
Pain management nursing advanced
    level. *See* Advanced practice pain
    management nursing
Parents. *See* Family
Patient
    assessment and, 4–5, 11
    collaboration and, 5, 28
    consultation and, 19
    defined, 35
    diagnosis and, 12
    ethics and, 29
    evaluation and, 21
    health teaching and promotion, 18
    outcomes identification and, 13
    planning and, 7, 14
    prescriptive authority and, 20
    professional practice
        evaluation and, 26

resource utilization and, 31
See also Education of patients
    and families; Family
Pattern theory, *v*
Pharmacologic agents. *See*
    Prescriptive authority
Planning, 5, 6
    collaboration and, 28
    consultation and, 19
    coordination of care and, 17
    diagnosis and, 12
    evaluation and, 21
    implementation and, 16
    leadership and, 32
    Nurse Practitioner and, 7
    outcomes identification and, 13
    standard of practice, 14–15
Policy. *See* Healthcare policy
Populations at risk for pain, 3, 7, 8
    See also Pain
Position statements, *vii,* 2, 3, 4, 5, 8
Practice environment, 5, 9
    collegiality and, 27
    coordination of care and, 17
    education and, 25
    leadership and, 32
    outcomes identification and, 13
    planning and, 14
    quality of practice and, 24
Practice settings, 7
Preceptors. *See* Mentoring
Prescriptive authority and
    treatment, 4, 5, 7, 8
    standard of practice, 20
Prevention of pain. *See under* Pain
Privacy. *See* Confidentiality
Process. *See* Nursing process
Professional development, 6
    education and, 25
    leadership and, 32

professional practice evaluation
and, 26
See also Education; Leadership
Professional organizations, 3, 9, 32
American Academy of Nurse
Practitioners (AANP), 7
American Geriatrics Society, 3
American Nurses Association
(ANA), *v, vi,* 1, 3, 4
American Nurses Credentialing
Center (ANCC), *vii,* 8
American Pain Society (APS), 2
American Society of Pain
Management Nurses, 1
American Society for Pain
Management Nursing
(ASPMN), *v–vi,* 1, 2, 4, 8
End-of-Life Nurse Educators
Consortium (ELNEC), *vii*
International Association for the
Study of Pain (IASP), *v,* 1
National Institutes of Health
(NIH), *vii*
National Center for Pain and
Palliative Care Research, *vii*
National League for Nursing
(NLN), 1
Nursing Pain Association, 2
World Health Organization
(WHO), 2
Professional performance. *See*
Standards of professional
performance
Professional practice evaluation
collegiality and, 27
education and, 25
standard of professional
performance, 26

Q
Quality of life, *v, vi,* 1, 4, 7
Quality of practice
Clinical Nurse Specialist and, 6
resource utilization and, 31
standard of professional
performance, 23–24

R
Recipient of care. *See* Patient
Referrals. *See* Collaboration;
Coordination of care
Regulatory and advisory
organizations
Agency for Healthcare Research
and Quality (AHRQ), *vi,* 2–3
Federation of State Boards of
Medicine, *vi*
Joint Commission on
Accreditation of Healthcare
Organizations (JCAHO), *vi,* 3, 5
Regulatory issues. *See* Laws, statutes,
and regulations
Research
Clinical Nurse Specialist and, 6
collaboration and, 28
implementation and, 16
in pain management nursing,
v, vi, 1–3, 6, 8, 9
planning and, 14, 15
prescriptive authority and, 20
quality of practice and, 23, 24
standard of professional
performance, 30
See also Evidence-based practice
Resource utilization
coordination of care and, 17
implementation and, 16
standard of professional
performance, 31

ANA NURSING STANDARDS PACKAGE

The set—totaling over 1,200 pages—contains the newly revised keystone publication of the set, *Nursing: Scope and Standards of Practice*, plus one each of the current volume for the 19 nursing specialty areas listed below. Each volume delineates and discusses the scope, status, and prospects of that specialized practice along with its generalist competencies, any advanced practice competencies, and the evidence-based standards with measurement criteria for practice and professional performance. **Pub #PKG**   *List $295 / Member $260*

The ANA Nursing Standards Package contains:

NURSING: SCOPE AND STANDARDS OF PRACTICE, 2004/168 pp. (*NEW EDITION*)
Includes the standards for clinical, non-clinical, and advanced practice, and the 1973, 1981, 1991, 1996, and 1998 editions.
#04SSNP   **List $19.95 / Member $16.95**

... plus 19 additional scope and standards of specialty practice.* All affordably priced at List $16.95/Member $13.45:

The latest additions to the set...

Nurse Administrators, 2004 (*NEW EDITION*) #03SSNA	Parish Nursing, 1998 #9806ST
Addictions Nursing, 2004 (*NEW EDITION*) #04SSAN	Pediatric Nursing, 2003 (*NEW EDITION*) #PNP23
Intellectual & Dvlptl Disabilities Nursing (*NEW*) #04SSID	Pediatric Oncology Nursing, 2000 #PONP20
Pain Management Nursing, 2005 (*1st EDITION*) #05SSPM	Psychiatric–Mental Health Nursing, 2000 #PMH20
Plastic Surgery Nursing, 2005 (*1st EDITION*) #05SSPS	Public Health Nursing, 1999 #9910PH
Neonatal Nursing, 2004 (*1st EDITION*) #04SSNN	
Vascular Nursing, 2004 (*1st EDITION*) #04SSVN	*Coming summer 2005:*

Coming summer 2005:
School Nursing: Scope & Standards of Practice (*NEW EDITION*)

... have joined these titles:

Diabetes Nursing (2nd EDITION), 2003	#DNP23
Gerontological Nursing, (2nd EDITION), 2001	#GNP21
Home Health Nursing, 1999	#9905HH
Neuroscience Nursing, 2002	#NNS22
Nursing Informatics, 2001	#NIP21
Nursing Professional Development, 2000	#NPD20
Palliative & Hospice Nursing, 2002	#HPN22

ANA STANDARDS STANDING ORDER PLAN
Great plan for university, hospital, and medical center libraries! Get the newest Standards as soon as they are published. We'll send the book along with an invoice. Plus, you'll save 10% off list price.
(*ANA members receive an additional 20% savings.*)
For details, or to enroll, call (800) 637-0323.

(* *Titles may be ordered separately. New and revised titles are being added continually.*)

ORDER FORM

Title	Price	Qty	Total
ANA Nursing Standards Package #PKG			
Shipping & Handling			
TOTAL			

Payment: (payment in U.S. dollars required)
[ ] Check enclosed (made payable to *American Nurses Association*)
Charge my [ ] VISA   [ ] MasterCard

Card # _____ Exp Date _____

Signature _____

Phone # _____ CMA# _____ **

****Your CMA I.D. number must be provided to receive member discount.*
20% discount off list price on orders of 20+ copies of the same title.

Shipping and Handling

	U.S.	Outside U.S.
Up to $25	$4	$8
$25.01–$50	$6	$12
$50.01–$100	$8	$16
$100.01–$200	$14	$24
$200.01–$300	$12	$32
$300.01 +	7% of total	15% of total

Shipping: 7 to 10 business days for domestic deliveries. 7 to 30 business days for international deliveries. Items cannot be delivered to a P.O. box.
All orders must include shipping and handling charges.

Ship to:
Name _____

Organization _____

Address _____

City/State/Zip _____

Phone # _____ Fax # _____

HOW TO ORDER
Online: WWW.NURSESBOOKS.ORG Phone: 800-637-0323 Fax: 770/280-4141
Mail: nursesbooks.org, P.O. Box 931895, Atlanta, GA 31193-1895